D1485617

Pocket Picture Guides

Ophthalmology

Colin M. Kirkness
BMedBiol, MB ChB (Aberdeen), FRCS (Edinburgh).

Lecturer, Department of Clinical Ophthalmology
Institute of Ophthalmology
Moorfields Eye Hospital
City Road, London, UK

Gower Medical Publishing · London · New York · 1985

© Copyright 1985 by Gower Medical Publishing Ltd.
34-42 Cleveland Street, London WIP 5FB, England.
All rights reserved. No part of this publication may be
reproduced, stored in a retrieval system or transmitted in
any form or by any means electronic, mechanical,
photocopying, recording or otherwise, without prior
written permission of the publisher.

Distribution limited to United Kingdom.

ISBN 0-906923-19-0

British Library Cataloguing in Publication Data
Kirkness, Colin
    Eye diseases. –
    (Pocket picture guide to clinical medicine; v.6)
    1. Eye – Diseases and defects
    I. Title   II. Series
    617.7   RE46

Project Editor: Fiona Carr
        Designer: Nigel Duffield
        Illustrator: Lynda Payne

Printed in Italy by Imago Publishing Ltd.

Contents

Introduction

It is impossible to condense the whole of ophthalmology into a few pictures, and inevitably by trying to do so distortions and bias are introduced. I hope that the reader will forgive these faults. If I have been able in this small guide to give a little insight into the fascinating field of eye disease then I will feel I have succeeded.

I am most grateful for the help I have received in preparing this Pocket Guide from the Department of Medical Illustration, Moorfields Eye Hospital, The Croydon Eye Unit, and Miss E. Eagling FRCS, Birimingham and Midland Eye Hospital.

Lids

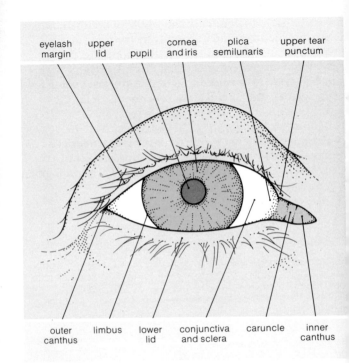

eyelash margin · upper lid · pupil · cornea and iris · plica semilunaris · upper tear punctum

outer canthus · limbus · lower lid · conjunctiva and sclera · caruncle · inner canthus

Fig.1 Normal eye.

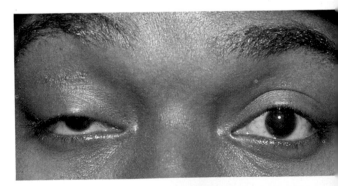

Fig.2 Ptosis. Loss of function of the levator palpebrae superioris results in ptosis, which may be bilateral or unilateral as here. Note the lid margin obscuring the pupil and causing amblyopia, the loss of the upper lid skin crease and the elevated eyebrow due to over-action of the frontalis muscle attempting to raise the lid.

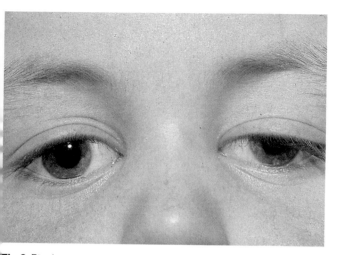

Fig.3 Ptosis - congenital. If there is congenital drooping of one upper lid it is due to defective development of the levator palpebrae superioris. If the lid obscures the pupil (i.e. the visual axis), treatment should not be delayed. Lesser degrees of ptosis can wait until the child is older.

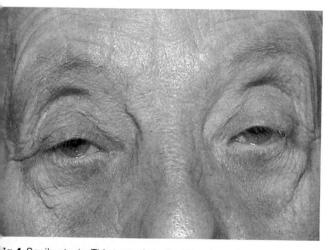

Fig.4 Senile ptosis. This type of ptosis differs from the previous examples in that it is neither due to maldevelopment nor paresis. In this case the levator aponeurosis has degenerated - 'levator disinsertion'. The frontalis can be seen to be overacting in an attempt to elevate the ptotic lid.

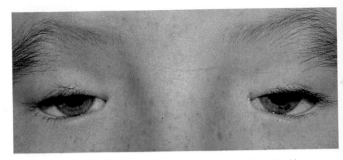

Fig.5 Blepharophimosis. This syndrome is usually inherited in an autosomal dominant fashion. There is a marked ptosis associated with a chin up head posture. Levator function is poor. In addition there is considerable telecanthus. A two stage plastic repair is generally necessary not only to improve cosmesis but also to prevent amblyopia.

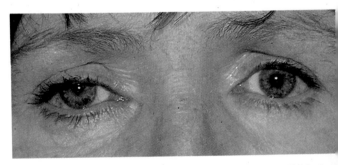

Fig.6 Horner's syndrome. The dilator muscle of the iris and Müller's muscle component in the levator are innervated by sympathetic nerves via the internal carotid plexus. Paresis leads to ptosis and miosis (unopposed parasympathetic action). If this is associated with loss of sweating locally (innervated via the external carotid plexus) then a classical case of Horner's syndrome is present.

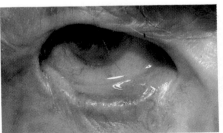

Fig.7 Cicatricial entropion. This eye has suffered severe burns to the surrounding skin and has an entropion caused by scar tissue distorting the lower lid, tethering it and pulling it away from the globe.

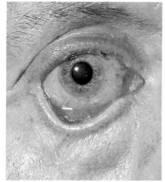

Fig.8 Ectropion. The ageing process in the lid leads to loss of muscle tone and absorption of collagen, resulting in lid laxity. The lower lid falls away from the globe, tears pool in the fornix and the exposed conjunctiva becomes dry, scarred and prone to infection. The medial canthal tendon may also slacken, allowing the punctum to move laterally. Proper assessment of this aspect is necessary prior to consideration of surgical methods of repair.

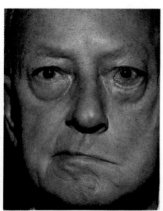

Fig.9 Ectropion - facial nerve palsy. Loss of tone associated with facial nerve palsy produces ectropion similar in nature to the senile type. Note the deviation of the mouth away from the affected side. Attempted closure of the lid produces upward deviation of the globe (Bell's phenomenon) protecting the cornea. If this response is lost, exposure and infection of the cornea may result. Note also the fleshy appearance of the thickened tarsal conjunctiva and the collection of mucus on the lashes.

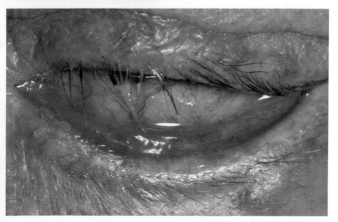

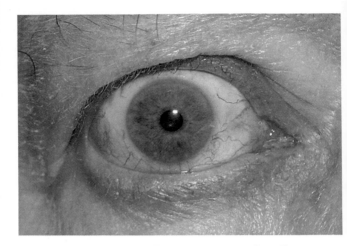

Fig.10 Dysthyroid retraction. Patients who have suffered hyper-thyroidism may subsequently develop orbital signs unrelated to their on-going thyroid state. In addition to proptosis, retraction of both upper and lower lids may be found. Lid lag may also be seen by asking the patient to look down: the lid follows the down-gaze, but only after an interval. Some cases may be relieved by guanethidine drops which block the sympathetic innervation of Müller's muscle.

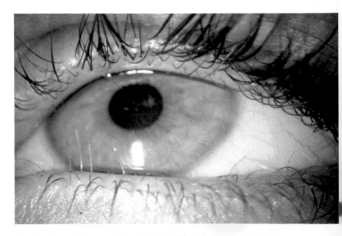

Fig.11 Dystichiasis. An extra row of fine lashes is present congenitally, usually in all four lids. The additional lashes arise from the openings of what would normally be meibomian glands. They point inwards, abrading the cornea, causing blepharospasm and photophobia.

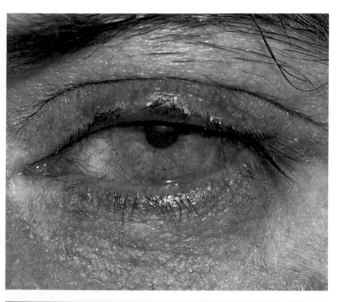

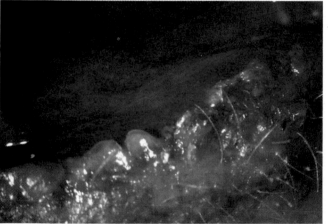

Fig.12 Blepharitis/meibomitis. The most common causative organism is *Staphylococcus epidermidis*. The lid margins and lashes become crusted and the fine vessels in the skin are engorged and telangiectatic; there is excess meibomian secretion. The meibomian glands may become infected (top). The lower picture shows a particularly severe form of blepharitis. The conjunctiva and cornea are predisposed to infection and immune reactions (marginal keratitis, see Fig.57 and keratoconjunctivitis sicca).

6

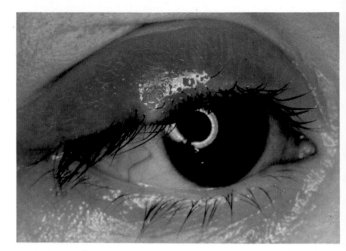

Fig.13 External stye or hordeolum. This is a pustule of a lash follicle caused by infection with *Staphylococcus aureus*. Reinfection is likely unless the organisms are eliminated from the surrounding skin.

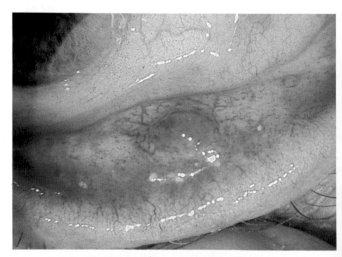

Fig.14 Chalazion. This represents one of the most common 'tumours' of the body. Sometimes wrongly called a meibomian cyst, it is a sterile lipogranulomatous inflammation of a meibomian gland. There is no cystic cavity. Granulation usually tracks to the conjunctival surface (as here) or may lie subcutaneously. Given time, many chalazia would absorb completely, but are frequently curetted.

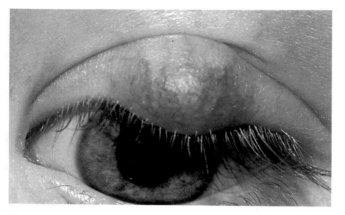

Fig.15 Haemangioma. This is usually congenital in origin. There are three main types of haemangioma: the port wine stain (naevus flammeus) is permanent, the cavernous haemangioma commonly found in the orbit does not involute, and the capillary haemangioma, as shown here, involutes but may at first grow alarmingly in size. There may be accompanying ocular and meningeal involvement.

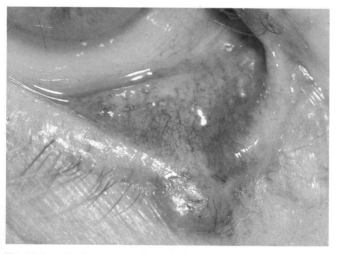

Fig.16 Basal cell carcinoma (rodent ulcer). These do not metastasize, but are locally invasive and more extensive than surface features would suggest. They arise commonly near the inner canthus and have raised, indurated edges with a central scale which may dislodge and bleed. Basal cell carcinoma is particularly common in fair-skinned people exposed to strong sunlight.

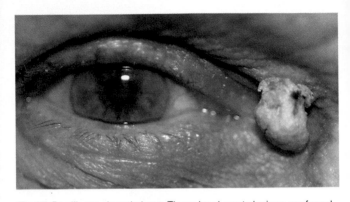

Fig.17 Papilloma - keratin horn. These hard, warty lesions are found in the elderly and grow very slowly. They are painless but may occasionally bleed. Despite their appearance, patients are often reluctant to have them removed.

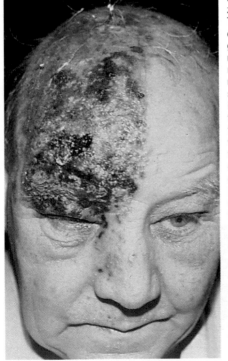

Fig.18 Herpes zoster ophthalmicus. The herpes virus lies dormant within the ganglia of sensory nerves and may be reactivated by a number of (obscure) stimuli. Pain occurs in the distribution of the nerve, soon followed by a vesicular eruption on the skin. If the ophthalmic division of the Vth nerve is involved, vesicles should be sought in the distribution of the nasociliary nerve (on the side of the nose). This implies that the eye itself will be affected with a more serious prognosis. III, IV, VI and even II cranial nerve involvement are occasionally found.

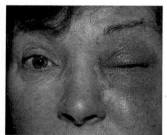

Fig.19 Allergic reaction. The well-circumscribed erythema and indurated skin usually present no problem in diagnosis. The conjunctiva is frequently oedematous and injected, and a history of local application of eye drops or ointment is obtained. A gradual subsidence of signs occurs with cessation of the exciting agent.

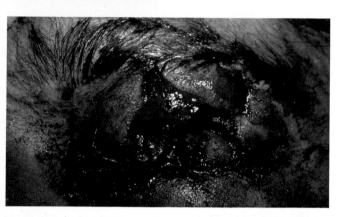

Fig.20 Trauma. Legislation making seat-belt wear compulsory has greatly reduced the number of such injuries. Here, broken glass has extensively lacerated both lids. It is imperative that the underlying globe is adequately examined, ideally under general anaesthesia, as a penetrating eye injury is highly likely.

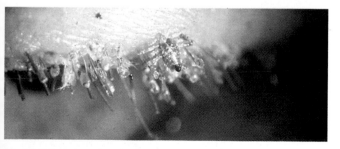

Fig.21 Infestation - lice. It is not uncommon to find the lashes infested with lice and nits. These are always *Pediculosis pubis*. Cutting the lashes may remove the nits and lice, but eserine drops paralyse them and ease their removal.

Orbit and Lacrimal System

Lacrimal System

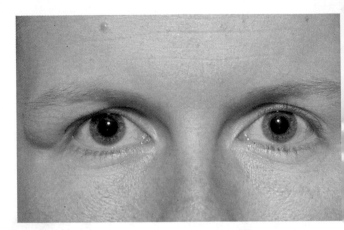

Fig.22 Lacrimal gland tumour. Tumours arising in the region of the lacrimal gland are most commonly benign mixed cell tumours, malignant adenocarcinoma or dermoids. The length of history is important as is the presence of pain and anaesthesia in the distribution of the lacrimal nerve. A short history with pain and an area of anaesthesia point to malignancy.

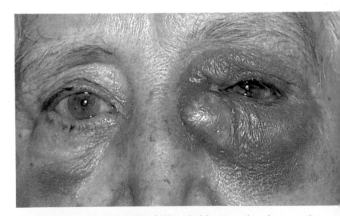

Fig.23 Acute dacryocystitis. Although this may arise *de novo*, the patient may have had an epiphora for some time, or even a mucocoele. The lacrimal sac forms a nidus for infection; an abscess develops and may point and burst - as this case is about to do. Note the surrounding cellulitis and that the inflammation has spread to the loose tissue below the other eye.

11

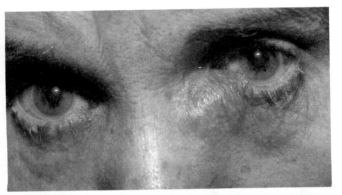

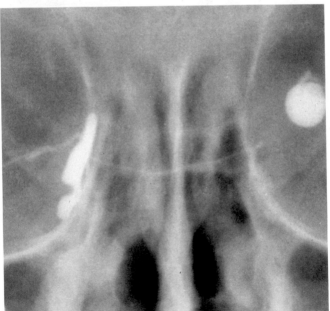

Fig.24 Mucocoele of the sac. This occurs in sacs which have suffered low grade infection which has been contained. The walls are atonic and the lumen fills with mucus which may be sterile. Pressure on the sac may express this mucopus via the puncta. A blockage of the lacrimal drainage system may be demonstrated by cannulating the puncta and injecting radio-opaque dye - a dacryocystogram (DCG) (lower picture). A normal sac is demonstrated (right) although the dye has not yet reached the nasal cavity. On the left, the blocked expanded sac is seen with blockage of the nasolacrimal duct.

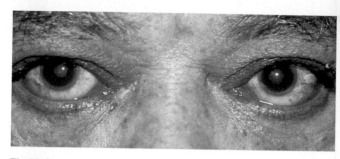

Fig.25 Proptosis. One of the earliest signs of exophthalmos is shown here. The inferior sclera is exposed and there is a gap of 2-3mm between the limbus and lower lid margin. This thyrotoxic patient did not demonstrate lid retraction but lid lag could be shown. The eyes felt sore and gritty, partly due to the exposure and partly to related changes in the tear film.

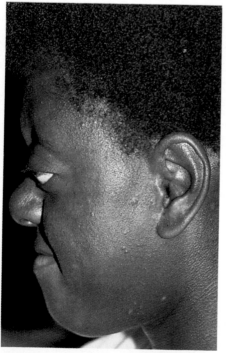

Fig.26 Pseudo-proptosis. An abnormally long eye (myopic) in a normal orbit, or a normal eye in a shallow orbit may give a false appearance of proptosis. In this case (Apert's syndrome), the orbit is shallow, the skull is flattened anteroposteriorly and the bridge of the nose is sunken.

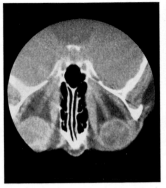
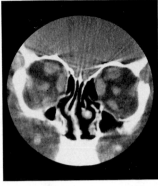

Fig.27 Dysthyroid eye disease. This is one of the most common causes of proptosis, whether unilateral or bilateral. The thyroid state may be hyper-, hypo- or euthyroid. Diagnosis was often difficult before CAT scanning was available to demonstrate the enlarged extraocular muscles, here particularly the medial recti. The infiltrated muscles become fibrotic, restricting movement and causing diplopia. The coronal views demonstrate the variable enlargement of all the recti muscles.

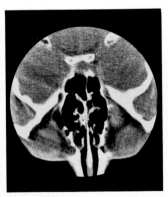
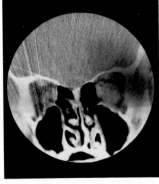

Fig.28 Optic nerve glioma. A unilateral proptosis associated with (progressive) loss of vision usually occurs early before involvement of the extraocular muscles. Computerised axial tomography has made investigation and visualisation of such lesions much easier. A large smooth fusiform swelling of the orbital portion of the left optic nerve can be seen (left). Glioma is by far the most likely diagnosis. It is worth noting that optic nerve gliomata may be an early manifestation of neurofibromatosis and other signs should be sought, especially in the young. Further definition of tumours may be obtained by coronal views (shown here).

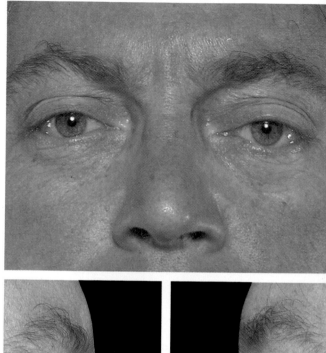

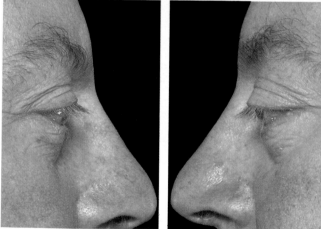

Fig.29 Proptosis (meningioma). Invasion of the orbit by tumours arising beyond it may also cause proptosis. The signs are subtle - a shallowing of the skin fold in the lid and a fullness below the orbital margin. Use of an exophthalmometer permits an accurate measurement of the degree of proptosis. In this case, a meningioma from the middle and anterior cranial fossae has invaded the orbit. The patient was only aware of some blurring of vision.

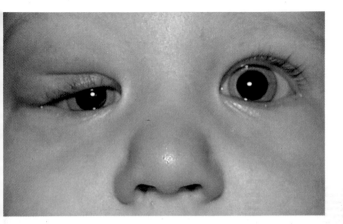

Fig.30 Dermoid. These are most commonly situated at the upper, outer part of the orbit but sometimes may extend more deeply into the orbit in a 'dumb-bell' fashion. This lesion is producing a mechanical ptosis but the visual axis is not involved and surgery may be delayed.

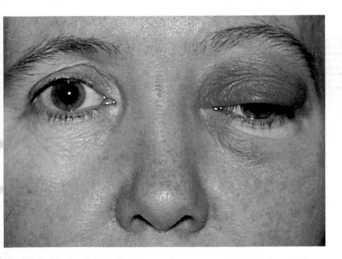

Fig.31 Orbital cellulitis. This is a serious, potentially lethal condition. The left upper lid is ptosed and there is a left hypotropia and exotropia. Oedema and erythema are present, limited in extent by the orbital septum. Often the infection has spread from an adjacent air sinus. Movement of the eye is painful. Diplopia may be apparent and proptosis, pyrexia and malaise may also be found. Vision is not usually affected until later, but immediate treatment is necessary to preserve vision and prevent intracranial spread.

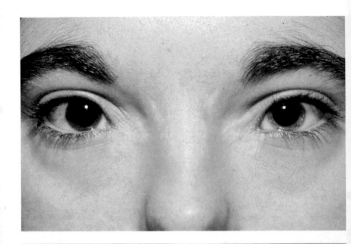

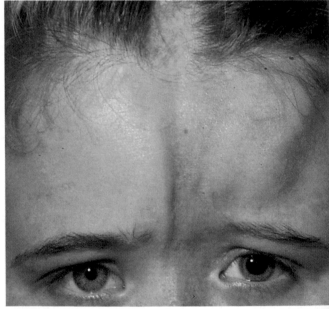

Fig.32 Hypertelorism. Widely set orbits are found in association with early ossification of the sphenoid and a number of maldevelopment syndromes. The intrapupillary distance and intracanthal distance is increased. This case (Waardenburg's syndrome) is associated with heterochromia and a 'coup de sabre' anomaly of the frontal bones (lower picture). Vision is usually unaffected.

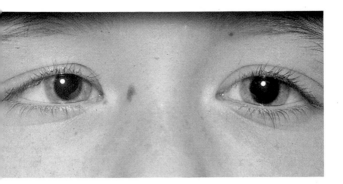

Fig.33 Convergent squint. Small degrees of convergent squint may be difficult to detect. Here, a light reflex is seen shining eccentrically in the cornea of the squinting eye. The reflex is shifted laterally because the eye is convergent. A refraction and fundus examination is mandatory before considering treatment.

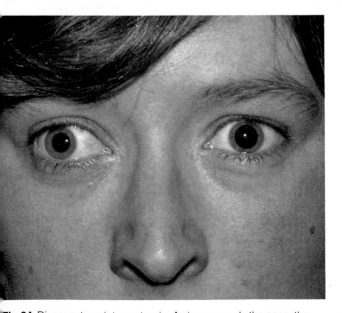

Fig.34 Divergent squint - exotropia. As is commonly the case, the diverging right eye is myopic and relatively amblyopic, in contrast with the normally-seeing left (emmetropic) eye. Divergence usually occurs at a later age than convergent squints. Eyes which become blind in later life generally become divergent, i.e. the eye which has poor visual input gradually takes up the position of rest.

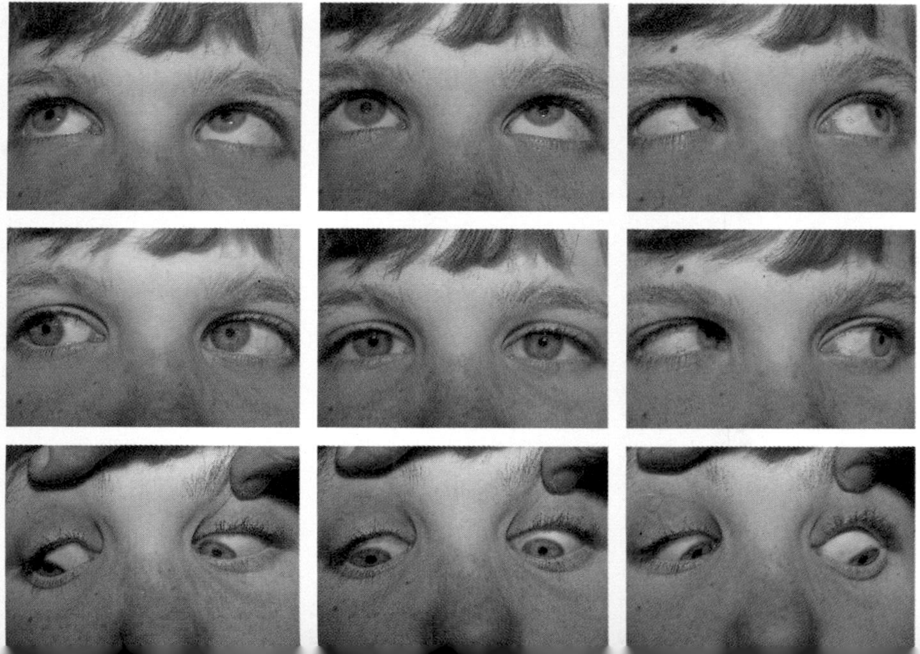

Fig.35 V-pattern esotropia. There is a left convergent squint which becomes more marked on down-gaze and less marked on up-gaze - hence a 'V' pattern - the eyes being more converged as they look down. On attempted adduction, the adducting eye drifts upwards. This is most frequently due to overactivity of the inferior oblique muscles.

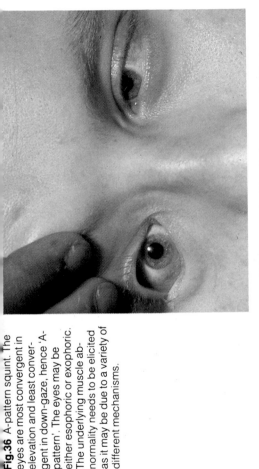

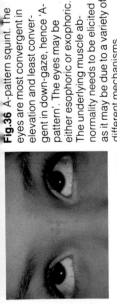

Fig.36 A-pattern squint. The eyes are most convergent in elevation and least convergent in down-gaze, hence 'A-pattern'. The eyes may be either esophoric or exophoric. The underlying muscle abnormality needs to be elicited as it may be due to a variety of different mechanisms.

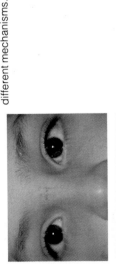

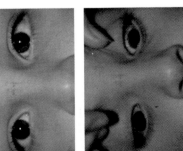

Fig.37 Third nerve palsy. The third nerve supplies the levator and all extraocular muscles except the superior oblique and lateral rectus. Here, the lid has to be elevated manually. The right eye is attempting to converge to match the left. It is hypotrophic and unable to adduct beyond the mid-line.

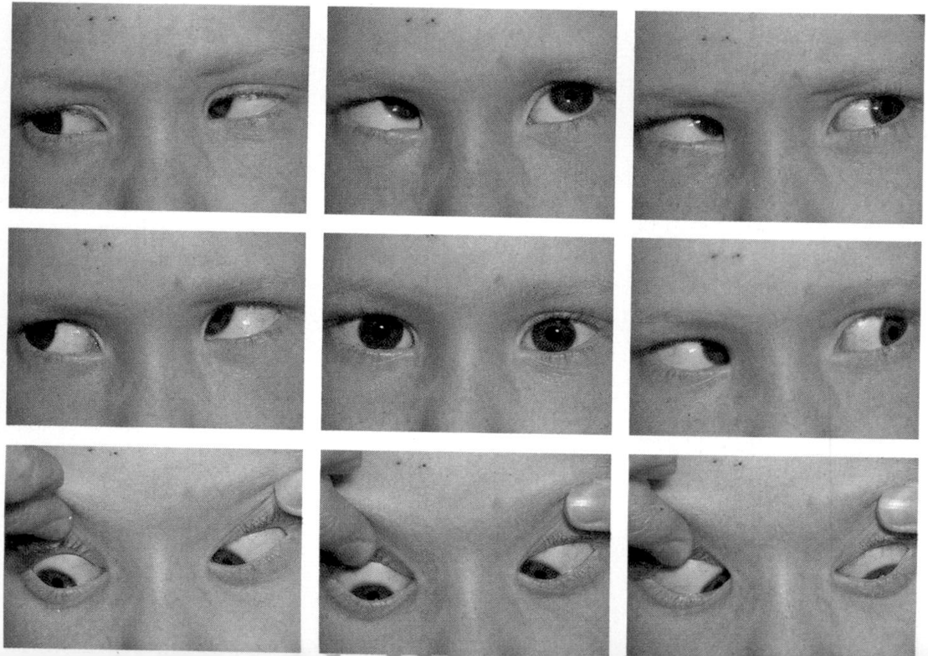

Fig.38 Fourth nerve palsy (underaction). This is a bilateral case and is associated with a small convergent squint. The action of the ipsilateral antagonist (inferior oblique) causes an up-shooting of the eye in adduction. In addition, adduction may occur on depression (inferior rectus overaction - ipsilateral synergist) and also abduction on elevation (underaction of superior rectus ipsilateral antagonist). Often congenital, this condition may be unmasked by a trivial event (decompensation) or it may follow closed head injury with damage to the medullary vellum.

21

Fig.39 Sixth nerve palsy (left). This leads to weakness of the lateral rectus. It may be congenital or can be caused by trauma, viral illness or demyelination. A small convergent squint is seen in the primary position with an inability of the eye to abduct. Bilaterality may occur, especially congenitally.

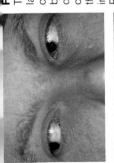
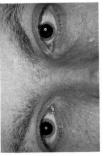
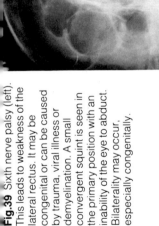

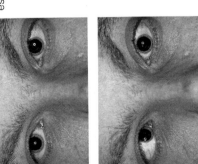

Fig.40 Blow-out fracture. Contusional injuries to the orbit may fracture either the floor (as here) or the medial wall, which are the thinnest parts of the orbit. Herniation of the contents of the orbit may be seen on X-ray. These are either fat or parts of the fibrous orbital septa which are attached to the muscle sheaths. Tethering of the muscle occurs (inferior rectus or medial rectus) producing a mechanical restriction of movement.
If the floor is injured, the infraorbital nerve may be damaged. Surgical emphysema may also be seen.

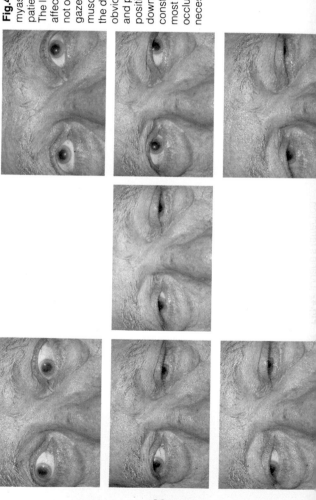

Fig.41 Incomitant squint - myasthenia gravis. This patient has a variable squint. The left eye is more severely affected; the squint varying not only with the position of gaze but also with time. The muscles show fatigability and the deviation becomes more obvious. Note the esotropia and ptosis in the primary position and the restricted down-gaze and up-gaze. The constantly varying diplopia is most disconcerting and occlusion of one eye was necessary in this case.

23

Fig.42 Duane's retraction syndrome. This is now considered to represent a mis-direction of innervation. The eyes are straight or slightly convergent in the primary position. Abduction is limited or absent in the affected eye. Adduction causes retraction of the globe and narrowing of the palpebral fissure. Observation of this latter point differentiates Duane's syndrome from a lateral rectus palsy and obviates neuro-logical investigation.

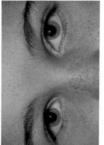
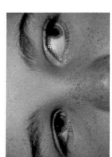

24

External Eye

Conjunctiva

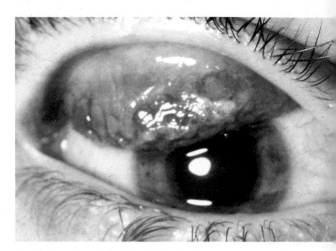

Fig.43 Vernal conjunctivitis. This allergic conjunctivitis is frequently found in patients with atopy. Giant papillae or 'cobblestones' are seen in the uper tarsus. The eyes are itchy, watery and accumulate mucus. Although more common in spring, cases may be seen at any time of year.

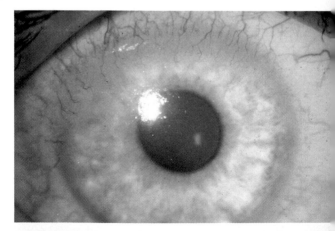

Fig.44 Pannus. Capillary loops and fibrous tissue descend over the cornea from the limbus, producing a typical pannus. In this case, secondary to excessive contact lens wear, the tear film and rest of th conjunctiva are healthy.

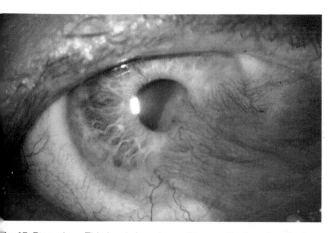

Fig.45 Pterygium. This is a 'wing-shaped' ingrowth of conjunctival-like tissue across the cornea, usually on the nasal side. The body extends far into the conjunctiva, up to or beyond the caruncle. There is an increased amount of vascular connective tissue - the collagen fibres resembling those found in pingueculae. The pathogenesis is complex, but they are often found in people living in dry, sunny climates. They are usually symptomless, but may affect vision if the visual axis is involved. Occasionally motility is compromised by tethering the globe.

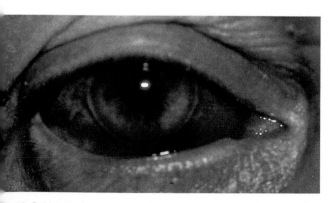

Fig.46 Subconjunctival haemorrhage. Rupture of one of the conjunctival veins allows extravasation of the blood into the potential space between the conjunctiva and Tenon's capsule. The cause is most often due to vessel wall fragility but occasionally hypertension and blood dyscrasias may present in this way. A sudden rise in venous pressure (a Valsalva manoeuvre), as in coughing or retching may produce multiple haemorrhages.

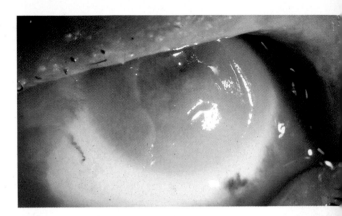

Fig.47 Burns. Burns affecting the external eye are more serious if large areas of tissue ischaemia result. This usually occurs in alkali burns where alkali penetrates the tissues, and rarely in thermal burns e.g. molten metal. This eye, shown some time after the injury, still shows nearly 90% of limbal ischaemia, both conjunctival and episcleral. There is a large epithelial defect and the induced enzymic (collagenase) activity is leading to disruption of the collagen fibres (corneal melting).

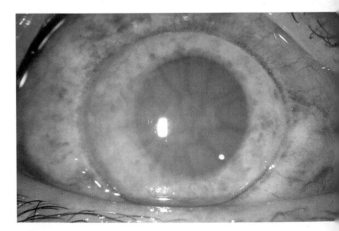

Fig.48 Alkali burns. Lime, sodium or potassium hydroxide or ammonium hydroxide and other strong alkalis cause severe chemic burns to the eye. Unlike acids, which coagulate tissues, alkalis penetrate deeply causing conjunctival and limbal ischaemia, endothelial damage, trabeculitis and cataract. Corneal 'melting' may follow. The end result is perforation or a severely vascularised cornea.

27

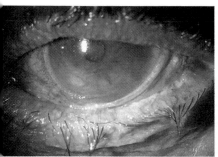

Fig.49 Benign mucous membrane pemphigoid. This inexorably progressive disease causes a cicatrisation of the conjunctiva; the associated loss of goblet cells disrupts the tear film, predisposing to infection. This eye has a large symblepharon extending up on to the temporal side of the cornea. The cornea itself has perforated at the eight o'clock position, although it is, as yet, relatively unscarred.

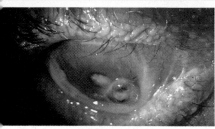

Fig.50 Stevens-Johnson syndrome (erythema multiforme et plurale exudativum). In response to an abnormal reaction to drugs (phenobarbitone, sulphonamides) or herpes or mycoplasma infections, a vesicular eruption occurs in the mucous membranes.Skin and nail beds may also be involved. This leads to conjunctival scarring, loss of mucus glands, corneal vascularisation and greatly reduced vision.

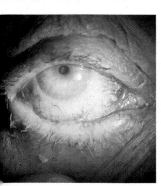
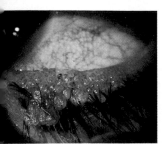

Fig.51 Papillomata. Infection of the conjunctiva with papoma virus results in papillomata, which may be sessile, as here, on the lid margin, or more frondlike. Treatment is difficult and apt to encourage spread. Cryotherapy offers the best prospect of eradication.

Sclera

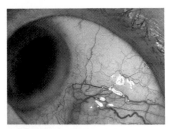

Fig.52 Episcleritis. This is a benign and usually self-limiting condition, although often very irritating to the sufferer. There may be an association with systemic collagen diseases. The deeper vessels of the episclera, lying on the surface of the sclera under the conjunctiva, are engorged in a patchy manner.

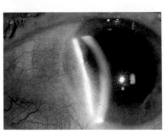

Fig.53 Sclerokeratitis. Scleritis differs from episcleritis in that corneal or uveal tissue may be involved in the inflammatory process. Ulceration is rare but the scleral collagen is commonly absorbed with resultant thinning. An underlying immune mechanism is commonly implicated.

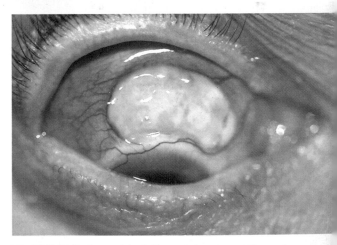

Fig.54 Scleritis (necrotizing). The anterior segment is most commonly affected. Severe or protracted pain is often present. A central necrotic area extends through the conjunctiva. The sclera becomes translucent and the underlying uvea shows through. Perforation may occur. Rheumatoid arthritis, polyarteritis nodosa and Wegener's granulomatosis are the most common underlying associated connective tissue diseases.

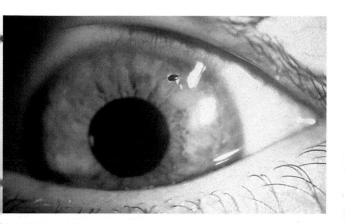

Fig.55 Corneal foreign bodies. These are common. If metallic, dissolution of the metal into the stroma may occur. Removal with a dressed orange stick or 23G needle is simple and effective.

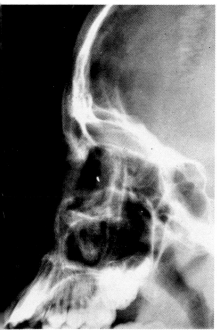

Fig.56 Intraocular foreign body. Any injury to the eye involving high velocity projectiles or unexplained trauma should be regarded as having a retained intra-ocular foreign body. Full examination should include X-ray, which will frequently reveal a retained intracular foreign body.

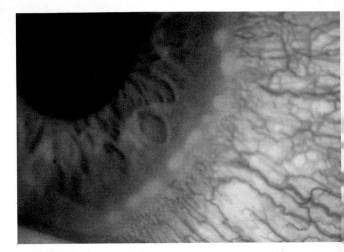

Fig.57 Marginal keratitis. Involvement of the superficial corneal periphery with localised conjunctival hyperaemia occurs as a manifestation of the allergenic response to bacterial toxins. One such toxin-producer is *Staphylococcus epidermidis* which is frequently overlooked as a potential pathogen.

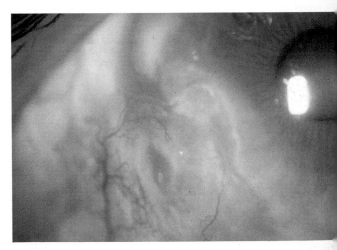

Fig.58 Rosacea keratitis. The guttering process that follows staphylococcal activity in rosacea tends to be self-limiting and rarely perforates. The cornea may remain thin at the periphery and is invaded by blood vessels in the superficial layers; these may leak lipid into the corneal stroma.

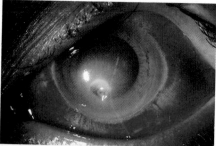

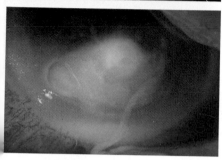

Fig.59 Suppurative keratitis. If infective organisms penetrate Bowman's membrane, e.g. following minor trauma of a foreign body (top), they are relatively free to multiply unhindered until leucocytes can invade the cornea, forming a corneal ulcer. An inflammatory reaction is also elicited in the anterior chamber in more severe cases (bottom) with more virulent organisms. The leucocytes settle out, forming a fluid level, hence the old name of hypopyon ulcer.

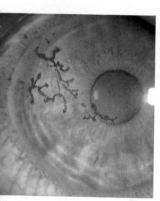
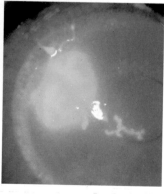

Fig.60 Dendritic ulcer (Herpes simplex). Another cause for sore, red, watery, photophobic eyes is herpes simplex virus. Viral infection of the epithelial cells rapidly leads to vesiculation and to breakdown of the epithelium in an irregular fashion as seen here. The abnormal epithelial surface stains readily with fluorescein, demonstrating the ulcer, which is difficult to see with the naked eye. Rose bengal may demonstrate the lesions (left). 'Satellite' lesions are common and may coalesce (right). *Steroids are highly dangerous in this condition (see Fig.62).*

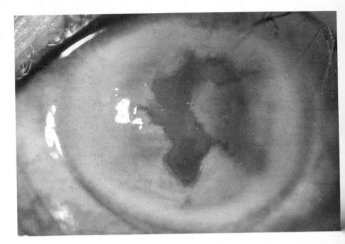

Fig.61 Amoeboid ulcer (Herpes simplex). Occasionally a dendritic ulcer becomes more virulent or aggressive and spreads widely, becoming amoeboid or geographic. Such ulcers heal slowly and may be the cause of much discomfort and subsequent scarring or thinning of the stroma.

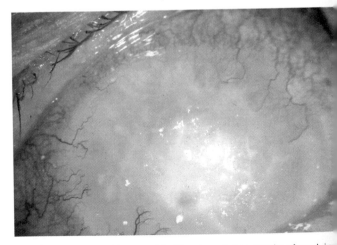

Fig.62 Herpes keratitis - steroids. The devastating results of applying steroids to a dendritic ulcer can be seen here. A severe inflammatory reaction occurs in the stroma following the exuberant viral activity. A large ulcer is seen superficially and the cornea is invaded by blood vessels. At best, a severely scarred cornea will result and at worst the eye will perforate and bacterial infection may supervene.

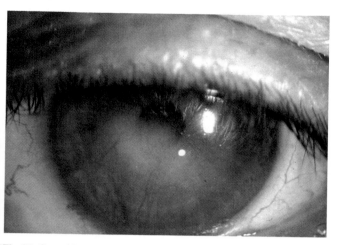

Fig.63 Corneal stromal keratitis. Certain infections, e.g. Herpes simplex, syphilis or tuberculosis, may excite an immunological reaction in the corneal stroma. The process may be slow and chronic or of acute onset but it induces corneal oedema and vascularisation, gradually obscuring vision.

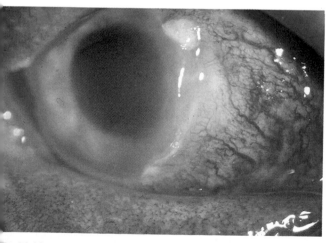

Fig.64 Mooren's ulcer. This painful progressive ulcer is rare, which is fortunate because it is extremely difficult to treat. It begins at the limbus as an area of infiltration which ulcerates and undermines the edge, thinning the cornea and spreading to involve the whole cornea, over several months to a year.

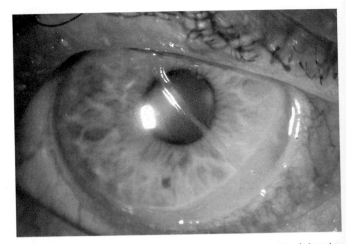

Fig.65 Marginal guttering. Several conditions produce a peripheral corneal ulcerative process which results in a 'melting' of the superficial corneal stroma. The ulcer appears to form a gutter around part of the circumference. Some cases are caused by coagulase-producing staphylococci, whereas others may have an immature basis, e.g. rosacea keratitis, rheumatoid arthritis, Mooren's ulcer and Terrien's ulcer.

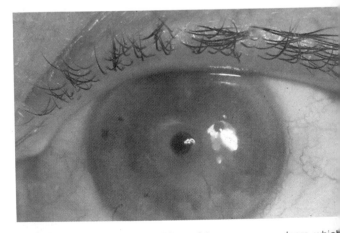

Fig.66 Descemetocoele. Conditions of the cornea, e.g. ulcers, which give rise to loss of stromal tissue may denude Descemet's membrane. As this is somewhat elastic, it herniates forwards under the influence of aqueous pressure. Perforation frequently ensues.

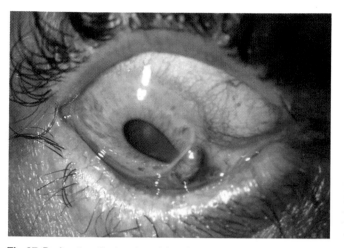

Fig.67 Perforation. Perforation of the globe may result from trauma or from a destructive pathological process, e.g. corneal melting. If the anterior segment is involved, the iris (or uvea and lens, if more posterior) may be seen prolapsing, causing distortion of the pupil. If trauma is the cause, a retained intraocular foreign body should be excluded.

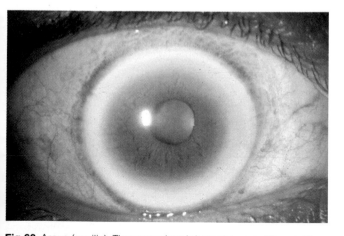

Fig.68 Arcus (senilis). The corneal periphery shows a diffuse infiltrate either in the form of an arc or (as in this case) a complete circle, due to lipid deposition in the stroma. It may be normal in the aged but if found in patients under 60 years of age it is advisable to investigate for hyperlipidaemia. Note the absence of blood vessels.

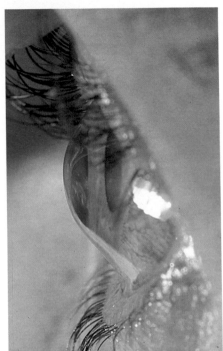

Fig.69 Keratoconus. In this condition due to abnormal lipid, the cornea becomes thinned centrally and assumes a conical appearance - an irregular astigmatism. Initially, this optical problem may be corrected with contact lenses but may eventually require penetrating keratoplasty.

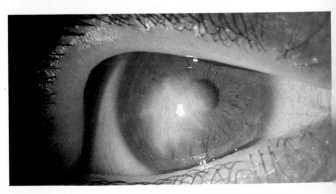

Fig.70 Acute hydrops. Splits or tears occurring locally in Descemet's membrane allow a sudden inrushing of fluid into the corneal stroma, producing a focal oedema, which persists until the endothelial cells can spread over and pump the excess fluid out. This may occur in advanced keratoconus (as in this case) and ultimately be responsible for scarring at the apex of the 'cone'.

37

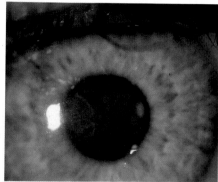

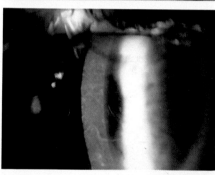

Fig.71 Dystrophy (Reiss-Buckler's). There are many corneal dystrophies, each affecting different parts of the cornea. Most are rare and many are hereditary. This is an example of an autosomal dominant dystrophy which affects Bowman's membrane. Irritation and discomfort begin in childhood and ring-like lines are laid down in the Bowman's layer (the overlying epithelium is unstable). The opacification progresses, but pain may subside for many years, until the condition is advanced. Good vision may be retained until late stages.

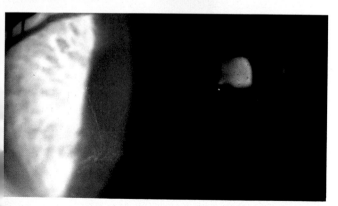

Fig.72 Cornea vorticellata (whorl-like dystrophy). Faint golden-brown lines are deposited in the upper layers of the cornea in whorl-like patterns. They are only seen with a slit-lamp, as an idiosyncratic response to drugs such as indomethanin, chloroquine and amiodesrone.

38

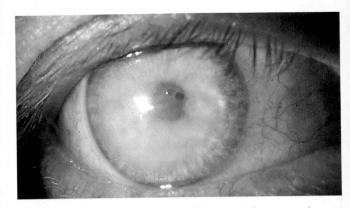

Fig.73 Bullous keratopathy. This condition results from corneal endothelial dysfunction. The healthy endothelium keeps the cornea in a state of relative dehydration and therefore clear. Dysfunction causes the cornea to become oedematous and ultimately epithelial vesicles or bullae develop. Intermittently these rupture producing an intense painful foreign body sensation. Two such bullae can be seen overlying the pupil. Visual acuity is severely reduced owing to oedema.

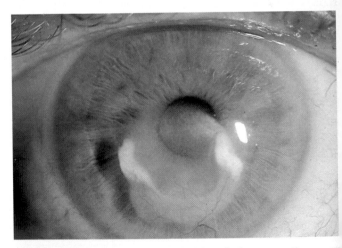

Fig.74 Lipid keratopathy. If new vessels invade the cornea, the capillary walls may allow transudation of lipids into the corneal stroma. The draining veins are usually easily seen but the feeding arterioles may be so fine as to be virtually invisible. The stromal opacity may reduce visual acuity considerably.

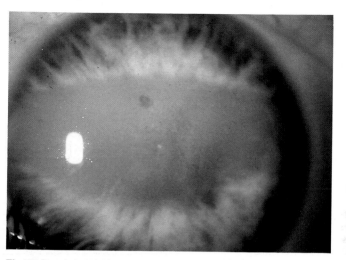

Fig.75 Band-shaped keratopathy. Long-standing disease of the eye, disturbing the nutrition or metabolism of the cornea may produce band-shaped keratopathy. Commonly found in blind eyes, it may also occur in iritis and corneal oedema. Calcium is deposited in the superficial corneal layers, mainly in the interpalpebral fissure.

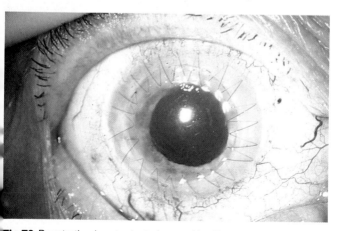

Fig.76 Penetrating keratoplasty (corneal graft). A full-thickness (penetrating) graft, transplanting stroma and endothelium, is now a safe and common operation to treat diseases causing corneal opacities. The transplanted cornea clears quickly (it becomes oedematous during cold storage) and a good level of vision is obtained at an early stage.

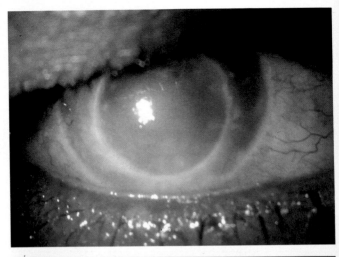

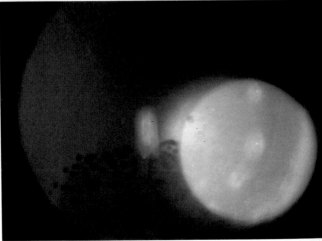

Fig.77 Corneal graft failure. Corneal grafts may fail for a number of reasons, but the most usual cause is the loss of endothelial cells. Although the cornea is immunologically privileged, it is not exempt and the endothelium can elicit an immune response, resulting in loss of function of the cell pump. Water enters the stroma and the graft becomes oedematous with progressive dysfunction. This may be either decompensation in a quiet eye or a suddenly active uveitis with a line of pigment and keratitic precipitates advancing on to the cornea with active iritis, i.e. rejection. The former is irreversible, the latter may be reversed by prompt treatment with intensive steroids.

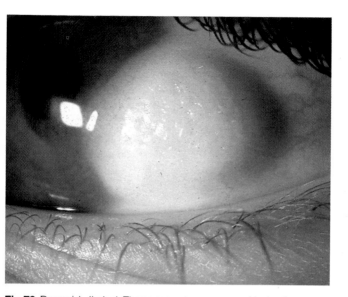

Fig.78 Dermoid - limbal. These are not uncommon. Nests of germ cells persist at the limbus or on the sclera. Skin, fat and hair follicles are produced. The lesion is unsightly, irritant due to the hair and keratin and may reduce vision by causing corneal astigmatism.

Globe

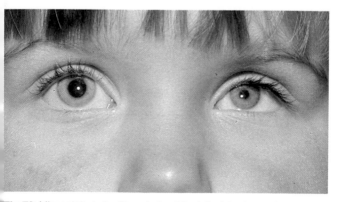

Fig.79 Microphthalmia. The whole of the left globe is small and vision is likely to be poor. Microphthalmia may be associated with a large number of other congenital abnormalities, but most commonly with congenital rubella.

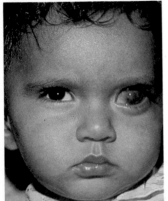

Fig.80 Buphthalmos. Failure in the development of the normal drainage mechanism produces an enlargement of the neonatal globe (left) (c.f. adult glaucoma where the globe is inelastic and the optic nerve is first to be damaged). The cornea enlarges but Descemet's membrane is less expansible and may split (the curvilinear lines shown here). This can result in corneal oedema. This second patient has stabilised and had good vision until cataract surgery was necessary. A broad iridectomy can be seen.

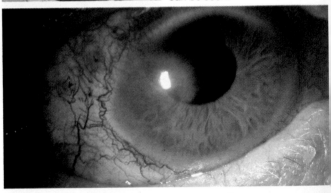

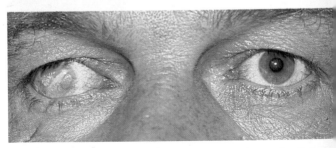

Fig.81 Phthisis bulbi. This man suffered a devastating perforating injury to his right globe, many years previously. The eye shows band keratopathy - calcium salts are deposited in an irregular plaque-like fashion in the cornea; the globe has become soft and has shrunk. The ciliary body becomes ischaemic, aqueous production falls, and as the globe collapses, the interior becomes disorganised and fibrotic.

Anterior Segment

Iris

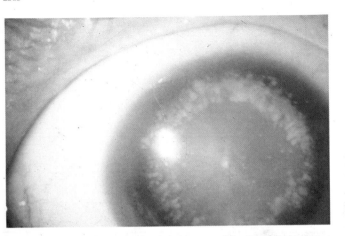

Fig.82 Aniridia. This is a congenital absence of the iris. Often some rudimentary iris tissue may be found. Anirida is hereditary and in some cases is associated with Wilm's tumour. Most commonly, vision is poor, there is nystagmus and glaucoma may develop. This case has cataract and the whole extent of the lens may be seen.

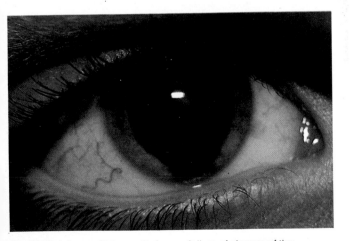

Fig.83 Coloboma. This results from a failure of closure of the embryological choroidal fissure. If only the anterior part is affected then an iris/ciliary defect exists. This may be associated with a coloboma of the posterior segment (Fig.84).

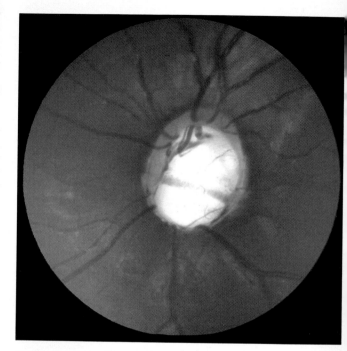

Fig.84 Coloboma. If the posterior part of the choroidal fissure is affected then a coloboma of the disc, macula, retina and choroid may be seen. Here, the superonasal part is normal, as are the vessels, but the inferotemporal part is excoriated and undermined. Here, the vision is poor because of the field defect.

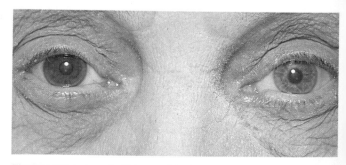

Fig.85 Heterochromia. This condition is usually more than a clinical curio. Either the darker or lighter eye can be abnormal. Probably the most common type is Fuch's heterochromic cyclitis, which is associated with cataract and glaucoma in the paler eye.

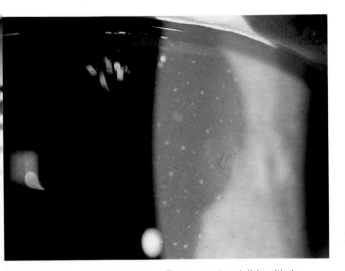

Fig.86 Iritis: keratitic precipitates. These may be visible with the naked eye if large, or may cause a dulling of the cornea, but most usually they require a slit-lamp for visualisation. They consist of collections of leucocytes or macrophages, adherent to the corneal endothelium and are an integral sign of iridocyclitis.

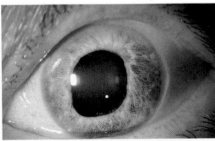

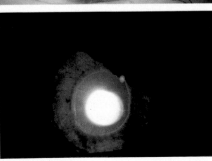

Fig.87 Iris atrophy. The two layers of the iris may be damaged by prolonged inflammation, e.g. iritis, herpes zoster or acute glaucoma. The pupil becomes fixed, dilated and irregular. Stroma is lost (here, nasally). Viewing the iris against the red fundal reflex shows windows of red coloration (transillumination) where posterior layer pigment is lost.

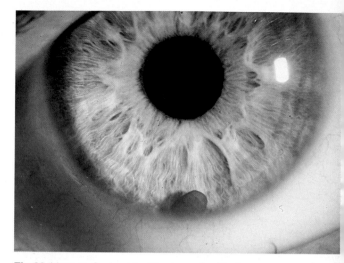

Fig.88 Iris cyst. Cysts of the iris pigment epithelium are not un-common. Often they appear at the pupil margin and may be mistaken for melanomata (see Fig.90). They are sometimes found secondary to using phospholine iodide drops. They may detach and float freely in the anterior chamber, as here.

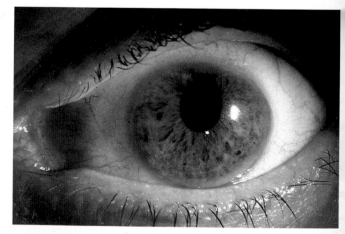

Fig.89 Ectropion uvea. In this condition the posterior pigmented layer of the iris has migrated or been drawn through the pupil on to the anterior surface. Iris tumours or any condition giving rise to fibrous membranes which are contractile (notably rubeosis iridis) may cause this condition.

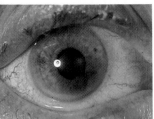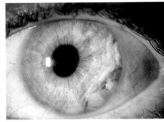

Fig.90 Malignant melanomata. The uveal tract is a common site for development of malignant melanomata. Those affecting the iris and sometimes the ciliary body tend to follow the path of least resistance and grow around the angle. They are often relatively benign, but may damage sight by blocking the angle and producing a secondary glaucoma. The clinical features indicating malignancy are actual increase in size, demonstrated by repeated photographic examination, nutrient vessels, the presence of satellite lesions, extension of the lesion into the angle and the onset of glaucoma, iritis or hyphaema. Precise diagnosis is sometimes impossible without histology. This tumour actually involves nearly 180° although only one quadrant appears to be affected.

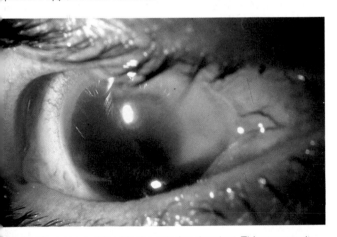

Fig.91 Hyphaema - blood in the anterior chamber. This may result from blunt trauma, surgical trauma, tumours or inflammation. The red cells settle and a clot may form, the distribution depending on the position of the patient's head. The aqueous outflow may be compromised and the intraocular pressure may rise causing discomfort and corneal oedema, as in this case. The vision is blurred to a variable extent. Spontaneous resorption usually takes place over several days without intervention, though reduced activity aids recovery.

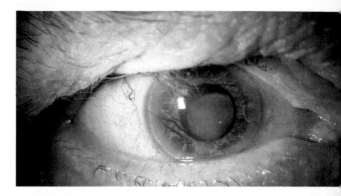

Fig.92 Rubeosis iridis. This is commonly seen in end-stage diabetes, or in other conditions in which there are extensive areas of retinal ischaemia. The induced neovascular process, seen here on the iris stroma, involves the drainage angle producing a secondary glaucoma and blindness.

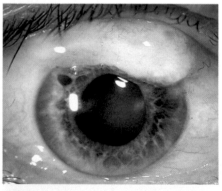

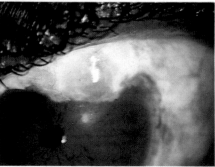

Fig.93 Filtration bleb. Many patients with glaucoma uncontrolled by medical therapy require filtration surgery to increase aqueous outflow and consequently reduce intraocular pressure. A small section of sclera and trabecular meshwork is excised so the aqueous can filter out through the remaining thickness of sclera under the conjunctiva, creating a small, localised bleb or blister. The bleb normally lies under the upper lid and causes no discomfort. Rarely, the bleb may become thinned and leak, or be predisposed to infection.

49

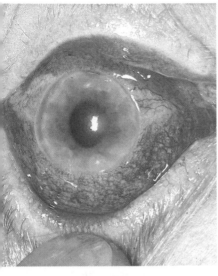

Fig.94 Acute glaucoma. Haloes may precede the development of pain and loss of vision. The pain may be prostrating and associated with nausea and vomiting. There is ciliary inject-ion, a hazy cornea and an oval, semi-dilated pupil. The eye feels very firm if not hard. The shallow-ness of the anterior chamber may be apparent. Hypermet-ropes in late middle age or older are most at risk. The other eye is also at risk.

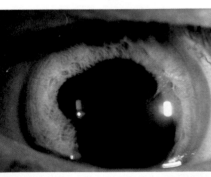

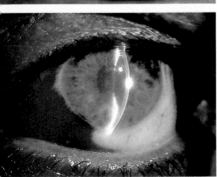

Fig.95 Posterior synechiae. Iritis leads to defects in the blood-eye barrier. Leakage of blood products into the aqueous allows the deposition of fibrin. At the pupil margin this will cause the iris to adhere to the lens. If not broken by dila-tion of the pupil soon after formation, the synechiae will become permanent and extensive. Ultimately a total ring synechia of the whole pupil margin will form, blocking the passage of aqueous which bal-loons the iris forwards. The intraocular pressure is elevated - iris bombé.

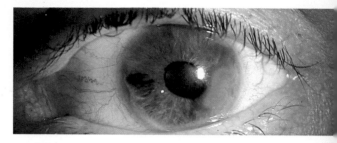

Fig.96 Irido-corneal endothelial syndrome. This includes a number of bizarre anterior segment syndromes which are probably all part of a spectrum. The endothelium shows patchy change with overlying corneal oedema. The iris is atrophic and often deficient and the pupil is irregular. Involvement of the angle leads to a secondary glaucoma. The condition is rarely bilateral.

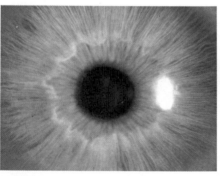

Fig.97 Albinism. Inability to form melanin results in albinism. In the more extreme forms the hair is white and the iris appears pinkish, due to blood in the iris and increased reflection from the fundus. Nystagmus is often present and the visual acuity is much reduced.

Lens

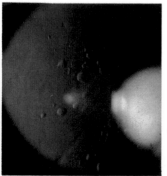

Fig.98 Cataract (posterior subcapsular). The nearer an opacity comes to the nodal point of the eye, the more profound its effect on vision. Thus an opacity at the posterior pole of the lens will have an exaggerated effect. Here a small plaque was enough to reduce acuity by 75%. By retro-illumination the changes can be seen to be more extensive.

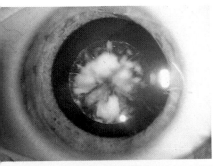

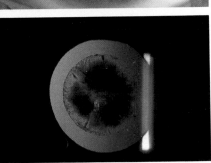

Fig.99
Lamellar/congenital cataract. As the lens is formed, concentric layers of lens fibres are laid down. Disruption of this process leads to loss of transparency and lamellar cataract; the more recent fibres laid down after the 'toxic' event are again clear. This is more easily seen by retro-illumination.

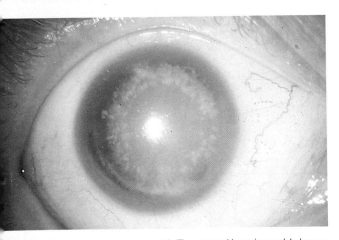

Fig.100 Cataract (nucleosclerosis). The central lens is muddy brown in colour due to the hard nucleus of the lens. In addition there are some cortical peripheral dot opacities. In this case, the whole cataractous lens is visible because the patient is aniridic.

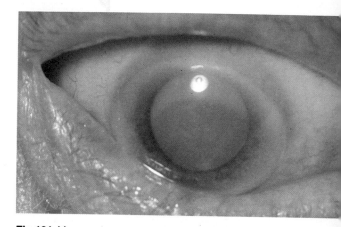

Fig.101 Morgagnian cataract. As the cataract progresses, the cortical layers may liquefy and the heavier nucleus (brown in this picture) sinks to the bottom of the capsular bag. The liquid fibres may absorb slowly, leaving a shrunken lens, or may leak through the capsule, producing a phakolytic glaucoma.

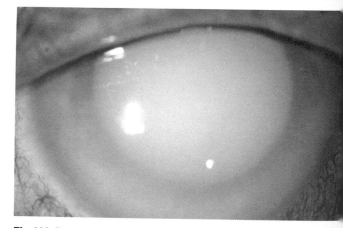

Fig.102 Phakolytic glaucoma. Hypermature cataracts may begin to show break-up of the lens fibres, so that the capsule contains a milky fluid and a nucleus which sinks to the bottom of the capsular bag. Leakage of the fluid material stimulates macrophages which engulf the proteinaceous material. These block the angle causing an intense glaucoma and corneal oedema. Small refringent crystals (of lens protein) may sometimes be seen in the anterior chamber.

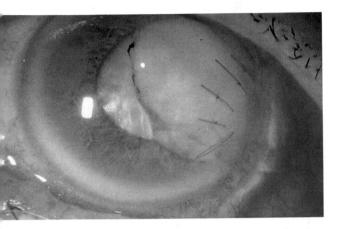

Fig.103 Cataract - traumatic. Penetrating injuries (and occasionally severe contusional injuries) are likely to damage the lens capsule. The lens fibres swell, opacifying the lens and occasionally extruding into the anterior chamber.

The corneal wound has been satisfactorily closed with nylon sutures, but a cataract has developed and will require removal urgently.

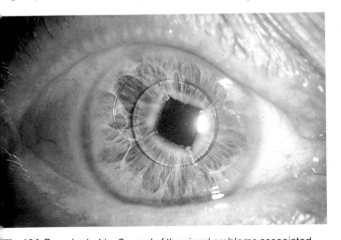

Fig.104 Pseudophakia. Several of the visual problems associated with aphakia may be solved by insertion of an intraocular lens at the time of cataract surgery. Many designs are available. Pictured here is a Binkhorst iris clip lens. The lens is held in place by the pupil, which becomes square-shaped. Such patients still may require glasses to correct presbyopia and astigmatism.

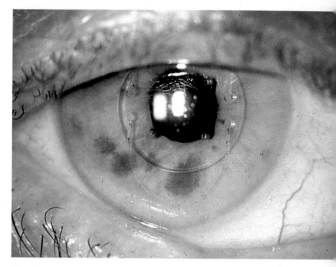

Fig.105 Iris clip intraocular lens. Two polypropylene loops lie anterio and posterior to the iris plane. The optic is situated anterior to the iris. The cataractous lens may have been removed intra- or extracapsular

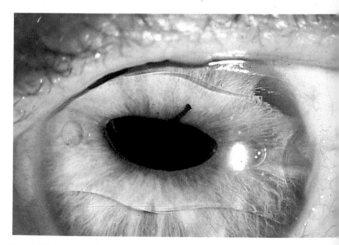

Fig.106 Anterior chamber lens. These lenses are produced from a solid piece of polymethymethacrylate or are supported in the angle of the anterior chamber. Though easy to insert, they give rise to many problems. The pupil may be oval or more seriously, the syndrome of uveitis-hyphaema-glaucoma (UGH) may exist.

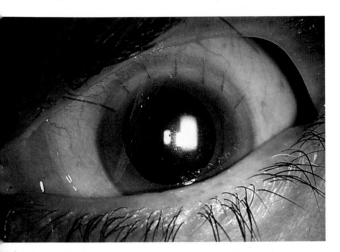

Fig.107 Pseudophakia - posterior chamber lens. The most acceptable method in modern cataract surgery is to perform an extracapsular lens extraction and to correct the aphakia by means of a lens set in the posterior chamber. These lenses are very much safer and provide the most 'natural' type of restored vision.

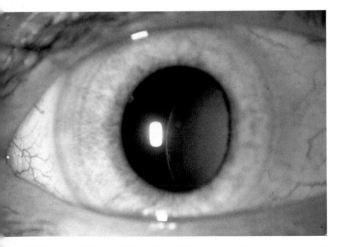

Fig.108 Traumatic lens subluxation. This occurs following trauma but may be a part of several syndromes, notably Marfan's and homocystinuria. The degree of subluxation varies considerably from rupture of a few zonular fibres to complete dislocation. Surgical intervention is rarely justified except in the case of pupil block. Some care is required to provide the best spectacle or contact lens correction.

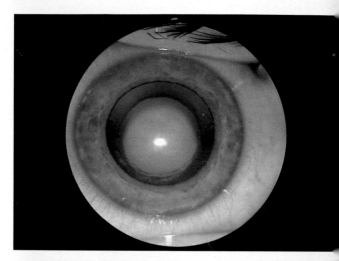

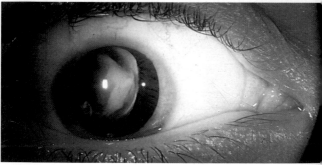

Fig.109 Leucocoria. Any white reflex seen through the pupil is called leucocoria. In adulthood, cataract or detachment of the retina are the most common causes; in childhood these may also occur, but a number of other conditions may be found, viz.

a Congenital cataract. It is important that all newborn babies be examined and that they be screened for congenital cataract. Delay in diagnosis and hence treatment may materially affect the visual prognosis.

b Persistent hyperplastic primary vitreous. This is usually unilateral. Instead of regressing, the primary embryological vitreous (which is vascular) persists as a whitish mass. Proper development of the secondary vitreous or retina is hindered. Such eyes are small and blind.

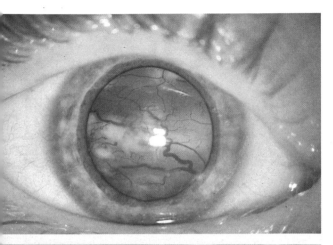

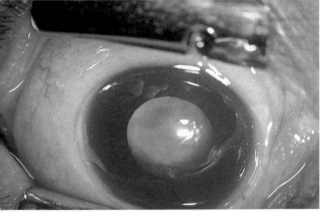

Retinoblastoma. This may be hereditary or may present spontaneously. In addition to leucocoria the child may present with a quint. There is a serous total detachment visible through the pupil and signs of the whitish tumour mass. Other forms may invade the itreous. Spread is direct along the optic nerve to the brain or occasionally through the sclera. Hereditary cases are usually bilatral. Spontaneous regression is occasionally found.

Retrolental fibroplasia. If the immature retina is exposed to excessive levels of oxygen, the blood vessels in its (growing) periphery are losed off. Subsequent reduction of PaO_2 causes a massive fibroascular response in the previously shut-down retinal periphery. This eads on to retinal detachment. Such a situation may be seen here. he incidence is currently increasing as more very low birth-weight hildren survive.

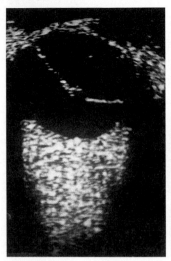

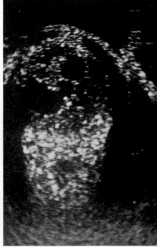

Fig.110 Posterior vitreous detachment (PVD) - horizontal B scan. Patients complain of development of floaters and occasionally some blurring of vision. The vitreous detachment is difficult to see and to photograph, but it shows up well on ultrasound. The posterior hyaloid echo can be seen crossing the sonically empty cavity of the globe. PVD occurs commonly in myopes and with ageing. The danger lies in the possibility of retinal tears being produced as the gel separates from the retina.

Fig.111 Vitreous haemorrhage. Symptoms range from a shower of floaters to sudden painless loss of vision. Dense vitreous haemorrhage obscures fundal details, preventing accurate diagnosis. Common causes are retinal tears, venous occlusion and/or diabetes. Ultrasound is most useful. Here, a funnel-shaped stippled area can be seen - this represents dense intragel opacity with the vitreous still tethered to the optic nerve. Venous occlusion is likely and hypertension and diabetes should be excluded.

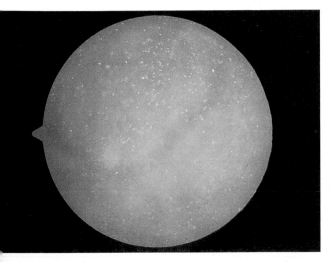

Fig.112 Asteroid hyalosis. This condition is usually unilateral and found in the elderly, but affects the vision only slightly. Spherical whitish round bodies of calcium soaps are mostly seen within the vitreous. It may be found in association with diabetes.

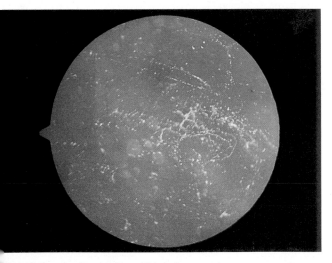

Fig.113 Synchysis scintillans. This is first seen in younger age groups. Flat, angular crystals of cholesterol move freely within the degenerate vitreous and fall to the floor of the cavity. It may be seen bilaterally and is usually secondary to trauma or prolonged disease.

Posterior Segment

Retina

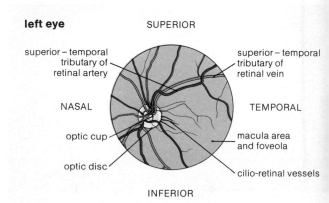

left eye

SUPERIOR

superior – temporal
tributary of
retinal artery

superior – temporal
tributary of
retinal vein

NASAL

TEMPORAL

optic cup

macula area
and foveola

optic disc

cilio-retinal vessels

INFERIOR

Fig.114 Normal fundus. The colour of the normal fundus may vary tremendously according to the amount of pigment present, from the very dark negro to the albino which has no melanin.

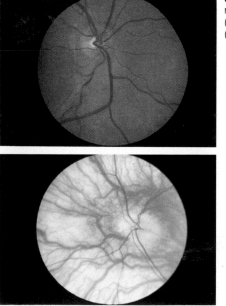

Fig.115 Normal negroid fundus (top). Albino fundus (bottom).

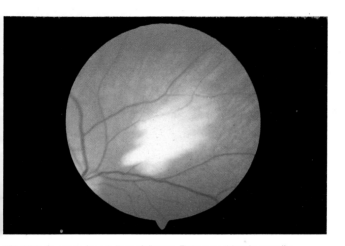

Fig.116 Opaque (medullated) fibres. This condition is usually asymptomatic and is discovered incidentally. Some retinal nerve fibres retain a medullated sheath and appear milky white, obscuring underlying detail including vessels. This patient's vision was unaffected and no treatment was necessary.

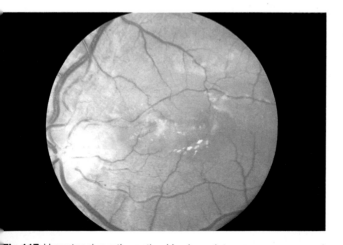

Fig.117 Hypertensive retinopathy. Hard exudates are seen surrounding the macula, beginning to form a star. There are a few nerve fibre layer fine haemorrhages between the disc and macula. Although there is no a-v nipping, the a-v crossing angle is nearly 90° and the veins are tortuous. Hypertension should always be excluded in such a picture, even in the young. This patient aged 20 had a BP untreated of 220/$_{160}$ due to polycystic kidney disease.

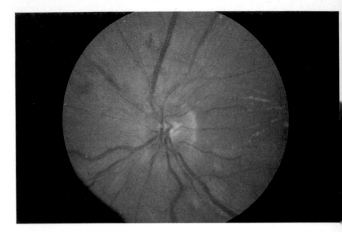

Fig.118 Malignant hypertension. There is papilloedema, although this is typically not very severe. The vessels are irregular and tortuous. There are haemorrhages and the edge of a macular star may be seen. 'Cotton wool' spots are developing. Accelerated (malignant) hypertension causes acute vascular damage and is less common with advancing age. Useful improvement of vision may follow successful medical therapy of the hypertension.

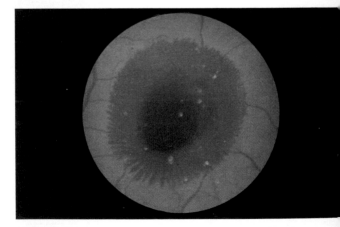

Fig.119 Subhyaloid haemorrhage. This usually arises from larger vessels at the posterior pole and lies between the retina and the vitreous. Often the blood cells settle, producing a fluid level with serum above. The haemorrhage may break through into the vitreous. Subhyaloid haemorrhage is an accompaniment of subarachnoid haemorrhage, although the mechanism is obscure.

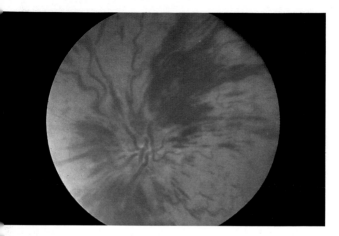

Fig.120 Central retinal vein occlusion. The disc is choked, with scarcely definable margins. The vessels, the veins in particular, are very tortuous and there is profuse haemorrhage in the nerve fibre layer. This is more common in late middle/old age. An underlying cause should be sought and treated accordingly.

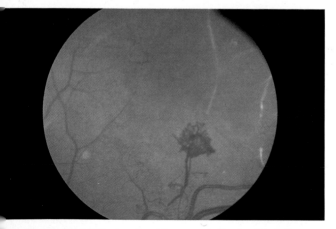

Fig.121 Vascular occlusion: late. The sequel of ischaemia in the retina is neovascularisation. Here the occluded vessels are obvious as white streaks. Proximal to this there is an area of new vessels and a dramatic 'sea fan'. These new vessels frequently rupture causing vitreous haemorrhages.

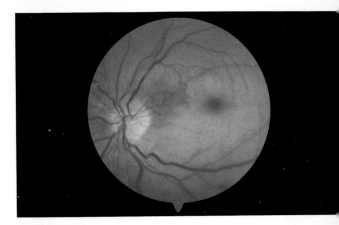

Fig.122 Central retinal artery occlusion. Occlusion of the central retinal artery produces retinal oedema. This has a milky appearance except over the macula, where the retina is thin, allowing the choroid to show through - the cherry-red spot. The arteries are thin and venous pulsation ceases. Occlusion is due to degeneration or embolism causing sudden blindness which will be permanent without treatment within two hours.

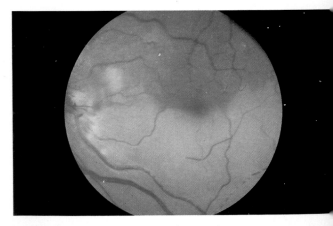

Fig.123 Branch artery occlusion. The occlusion of the retinal artery may spare some branches, producing only a branch artery occlusion. In this instance, the retinal oedema is solely in the area of distribution of the affected vessel. 'Cattle-trucking' of the stagnant blood column can be seen clearly.

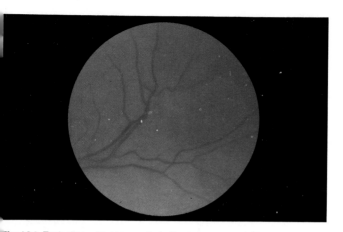

Fig.124 Embolism. Blockage of a retinal artery may be caused by an embolus (Hollenhorst plaque) either from a valvular vegetation or atheromatous plaque. Commonly these give rise to amaurosis fugax (temporary blindness). Because this plaque is flat it will allow blood flow on either side, despite being wedged in a vessel. It may, of course, block a vessel by lying across the lumen. Investigation and treatment of sources may prevent further episodes.

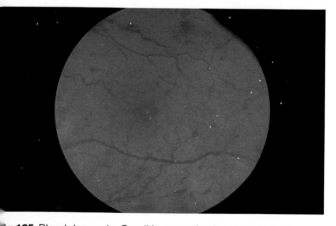

Fig.125 Blood dyscrasia. Conditions causing increased blood viscosity may affect the retina. Both multiple myeloma and Waldenström's macroglobulinaemia may cause retinal venous budging and occlusion with scattered haemorrhages. The veins may be irregular, resembling a string of sausages. Treatment of the underlying condition may produce dramatic resolution of the fundal appearances.

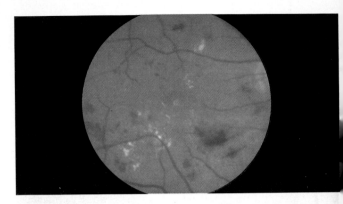

Fig.126 Diabetic background retinopathy. The very earliest sign of microaneuryms has given way to dot and blot haemorrhages and hard exudates. The lesions are scattered but the fovea is spared and vision is still good. The basic pathology is capillary under perfusion, and the condition will progress to one of the most advanced forms of retinopathy.

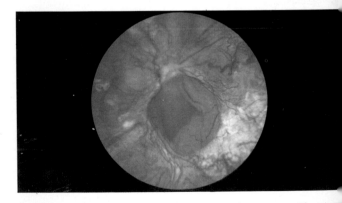

Fig.127 Diabetes: retinal traction detachment. In severe proliferative diabetic retinopathy the end stage is traction retinal detachment. Contractile elements in the fibrovascular proliferative membrane pull on the retina, distorting and finally detaching it. The retina is rigid and relatively immobile; there is little, if any, subretinal fluid and a hole (if found at all) is secondary in nature. The patient will complain of reduced or distorted vision of sudden or rapid onset. It is important to recognise and treat ischaemic areas in the retina before the neo-vascularisation has reached this stage. Fundal examination under mydriasis should be regularly performed on diabetics even in the absence of visual complaints.

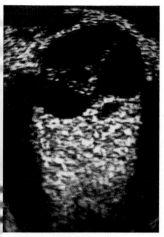

Fig.128 Traction detachment. Frequently such eyes have opacities in the media, e.g. cataract/vitreous haemorrhage. Ultrasound again plays a useful role. Here, in a very similar case to Fig.127, the gel can be seen partially detached but inserting into an elevated portion of retina at the posterior pole. The posterior hyaloid echo is linear, indicating that it is under tension (it would also appear rigid on dynamic views). There is, in addition, a small amount of intergel opacity which would limit fundal visualisation.

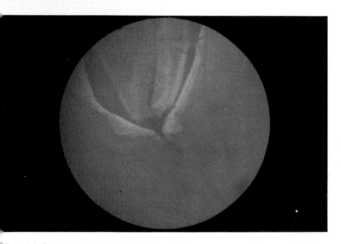

Fig.129 Retinal detachment: U-tear. The presence of a tear or hole in the retina predisposes to rhegmatogenous retinal detachment. Vitreous traction upon an area of 'weak' peripheral retina results in a U-shaped tear, the flap or operculum of which has a base pointing to the periphery. Continued vitreous traction allows fluid to track under the retina causing detachment. It may be symptomless but often is associated with 'flashing lights' or floaters. Here the U-tear shows signs of the edges elevating (i.e. detachment just starting). The pigmented line indicates abnormal vitreo-retinal adhesion. Blood vessels may be seen crossing the tear - if these break vitreous haemorrhage will ensue. Full papillary dilation is necessary to adequately examine for such condition.

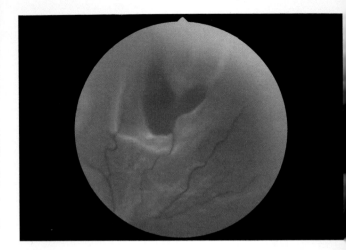

Fig.130 Retinal detachment: bulla with tear. Following the formation of a tear, fluid has entered the subretinal space, detaching the retina, which has lost its normal reflex becoming greyish or opalescent with a finely wrinkled surface. Such a bulla is mobile and floppy, encouraging extension of the detachment. A field defect corresponding to the area detached will be found, central vision being lost when the macula is involved. The exact distribution depends on the position of the tear, gravity being important in determining the spread of subretinal fluid. The patient may describe a 'curtain' or 'shutter' coming across the field of vision. It is painless.

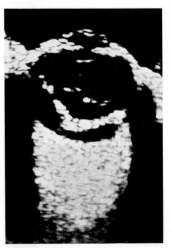

Fig.131 Retinal detachment: horizontal B scan. The haemorrhage that sometimes accompanies tear formation may also obscure the subsequent retinal detachment. Here, two linear echoes are seen in the cavity. The finer, more anterior echo represents the detached posterior vitreous which contains poorly shown opacity; the thicker more posterior echo represents the detached retina. Such information is invaluable in determining the urgency for surgery.

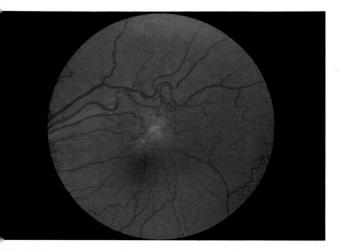

Fig.132 Macular pucker. The formation of epiretinal membranes induces the proliferation of myoepithelial cells. These contract as they mature, distorting the retina, and if extensive may lead to traction retinal detachment. They may avulse spontaneously.

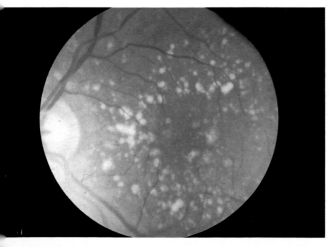

Fig.133 Colloid bodies or drusen. These are tiny yellowish discrete lesions at the levels of Bruch's membrane. They may become confluent if profuse. They are degenerate pigment epithelium cells. They may be found alone with normal vision or may be found in the presence of reduced vision in senile macular degeneration or disciform degeneration of the macula.

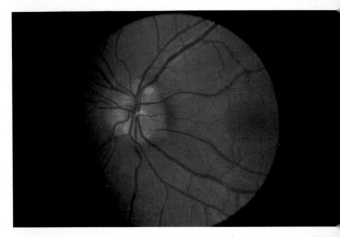

Fig.134 Papilloedema. The outline of the disc is becoming obscured and the cup is filling in. The nerve head begins to swell above the surface of the retina. Flame-shaped haemorrhages are seen and the veins are distended. The normal blind spot is enlarged and may extend towards the central macular area. Immediate investigation is essential.

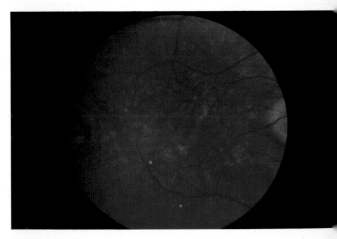

Fig.135 Senile macular degeneration. One of the major causes of blindness in the elderly, this condition presents as early stippling followed by the appearance of gross pigment clumps and drusen (colloid bodies). The visual loss is often profound and usually greater than the fundal appearance would indicate.

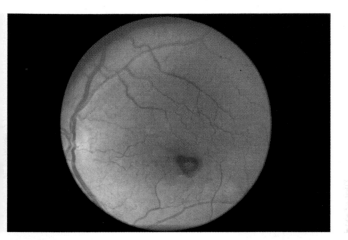

Fig.136 Macular haemorrhage. Haemorrhage at the macula (or elsewhere in the retina) may be due to hypertension diabetes, blood dyscrasia or intrinsic eye disease such as disciform degeneration or Fuch's spot in myopia. In any case investigation is warranted.

Macula

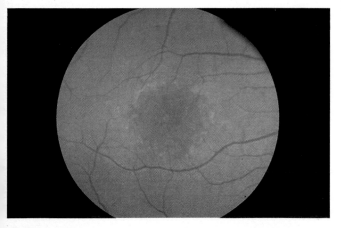

Fig.137 Hereditary macular dystrophies (Stargardt's disease). A number of hereditary macular dystrophies exist, primarily affecting the pigment epithelium and underlying choriocapillaris. The condition is usually 'dry', lacking oedema or exudation and treatment is limited. Presentation is in early adulthood with reduced or distorted vision, although useful acuity may be preserved for many years.

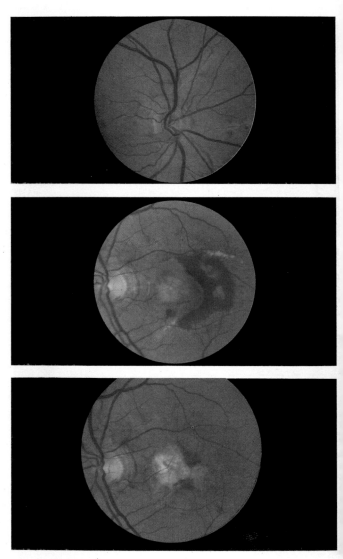

Fig.138 Angioid streaks. This is a rare condition occurring in middle age and usually affecting the macula. The colour of the streaks varies even in the same patient. Bruch's membrane is degenerate and there is a predisposition to disciform formation. They may be associated with Ehlers-Danlos syndrome, Paget's disease and a number of rarer conditions.

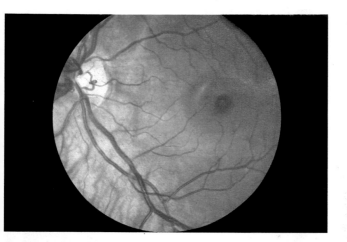

Fig.139 Solar eclipse burn. A complaint of visual loss or scotoma following observation of the sun or a solar eclipse through inadequate protection is unfortunately relatively common. The only abnormality is a discrete 'punched out' area at, or near, the fovea. Later pigmentary change may be seen. Commonly these unfortunates are amblyopic and the dominant is so affected.

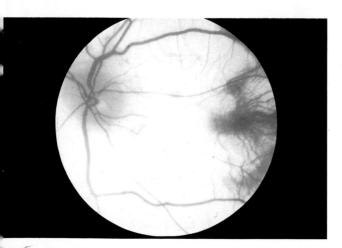

Fig.140 Choroidiremia. This X-linked hereditary tapetoretinal degeneration presents with night-blindness, visual field constriction and loss of acuity. Pigment mottling may be found, but unlike retinitis pigmentosa (Fig.141) it does not invade the retina. Female carriers may exhibit a very much milder form of the condition.

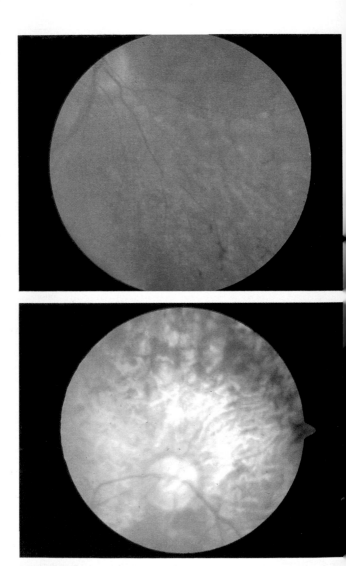

Fig.141 Retinitis pigmentosa. This is a progressive hereditary condition (the mode of inheritance varies in different pedigrees). It presents with night-blindness and advances to constricted visual fields and loss of acuity. By the time the typical findings of bone corpuscle pigmentation advancing centrally, attenuation of vessels, and optic atrophy are seen, visual loss is profound. The condition is untreatable.

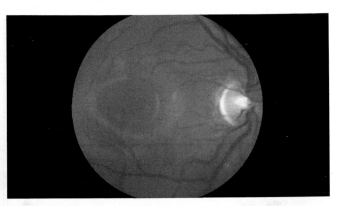

Fig.142 Central serous retinopathy. Ophthalmoscopy reveals a blurred foveal reflex with a circular or oval raised area surrounding the fovea. This is caused by an accumulation of serous fluid subretinally through an underlying pigment epithelium defect. Fine yellowish dots may be seen within the area and cystic changes may develop if long-standing. There is usually only a slight loss in visual acuity and distortion of lines in young to early middle-aged males. Resolution occurs over a few weeks but relapses occur in one third of patients.

Choroid

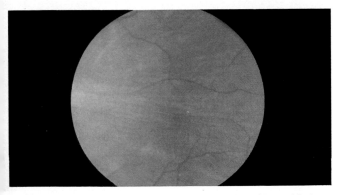

Fig.143 Choroidal folds. In conditions in which there is an orbital mass, choroidal folds may be seen, due to distortion of the globe and the choroid. If the macular area is involved, acuity may be affected. The folds resolve if the underlying cause is removed. Unfortunately their presence is unhelpful diagnostically.

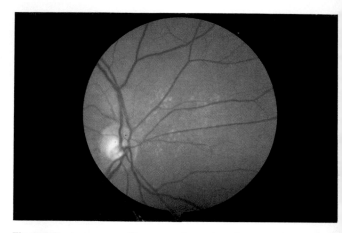

Fig.144 Benign naevus. These naevi are often discovered incidentally and are a great source of anxiety because their main differential diagnosis is from malignant melanoma. The presence of drusen on the surface indicates a benign lesion, probably long-standing. Long-term follow-up with serial photography may demonstrate lack of growth, but no one test is entirely reliable.

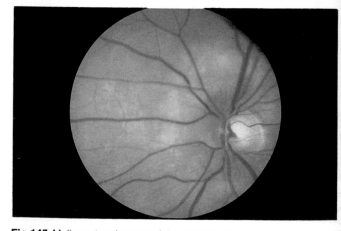

Fig.145 Malignant melanoma of the choroid. The choroid is a frequent site for malignant melanoma development. Diagnosis may often prove difficult. This fundus shows a greyish elevation surrounding the retina. The vessels at the disc can be seen climbing over the mass. In effect, there is a solid retinal detachment. Lateral stages may show subretinal accumulation of serous fluid. Good vision may be preserved for some time.

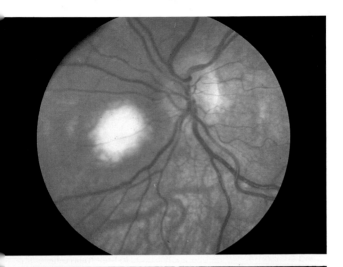

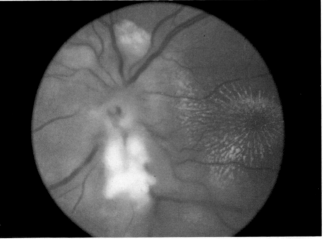

Fig.146 Choroiditis. A complaint of slightly blurred vision, sometimes with floaters, is often the presentation. There may be a mild anterior uveitis and cells may appear in the vitreous. A slightly raised whitish patch with blurred edges is present. They usually lie at the posterior pole and may be multiple.

As the inflammation progresses or subsides, the edges become pigmented and the chorioretina atrophies in that area. If situated at the macula, visual acuity will be lost; if elsewhere, the effect is minimal. The causative agent is frequently toxoplasma, but histoplasmosis and toxocara may give a similar picture.

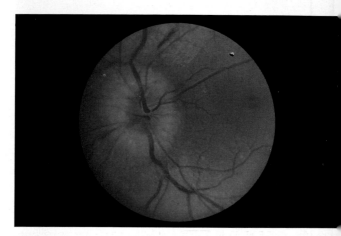

Fig.147 Papilloedema. The normal blind spot is enlarged and may extend towards the central macular area. In later stages the disc becomes pinker or greyish red, approximating to the colour of the surrounding retina. The venous blood column appears darker and retinal haemorrhages may be profuse, occasionally even becoming subhyaloid. Retinal exudates are sometimes seen.

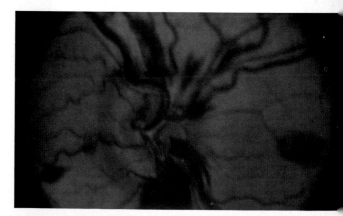

Fig.148 Papilloedema. The outline of the disc is becoming obscured and the cup is filling in. The nerve head begins to swell above the surface of the retina. Flame-shaped haemorrhages are seen and the veins are distended. Immediate investigation is essential.

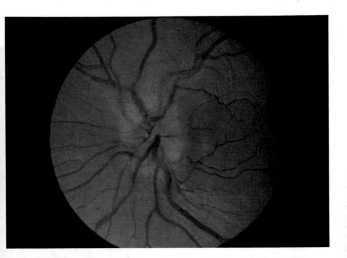

Fig.149 Optic neuritis. In its most florid form, this may be indistinguishable from papilloedema. At the other extreme, in retrobulbar neuritis the nerve head may be normal. The vision is vastly reduced, colour discrimination is poor and pain on movement may follow. There is a relative afferent papillary defect and a central or paracentral scotoma. Multiple sclerosis is the most common underlying condition.

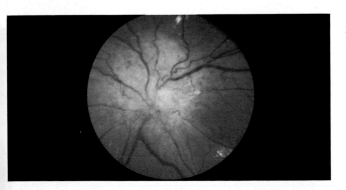

Fig.150 Ischaemic papillopathy. Ischaemic papillopathy is due to microvascular occlusion in the nerve head. Abrupt loss of vision in the middle-aged and elderly is the presentation, due to cranial arteritis or arteriosclerosis. The disc is moderately swollen and pale; a few linear haemorrhages may be seen. Other evidence of arteriosclerosis (e.g. hard exudates, as here) may be seen. Optic atrophy eventually occurs. Pain and raised ESR is diagnostic of cranial arteritis. Systemic steroids are mandatory.

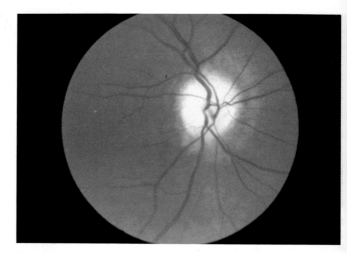

Fig.151 Ischaemic papillopathy (late). Optic atrophy inevitably follows a ischaemic episode. The disc is pale and featureless. The visual loss is profound and little if any recovery takes place.

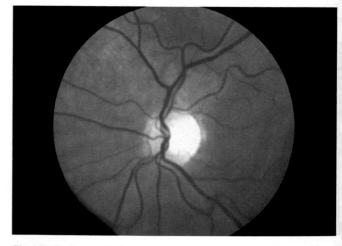

Fig.152 Optic atrophy (optic nerve compression). The only feature is visual loss (acuity and field); pain and headache, if present, occur late as do the disc appearances. The disc is sharply demarcated, pale and featureless. Field defect is of paramount importance. The initial central scotoma spreads peripherally to a small peripheral rim before that too is lost with total blindness. Compression is by a meningioma or, most commonly, unsuspected aneurysm of the nerve.

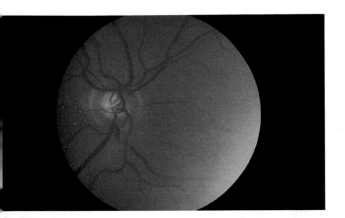

Fig.153 Glaucomatous cupping (early) - raised intraocular pressure. Initially, in patients with chronic simple glaucoma, the vision is normal and an early field defect can only be detected with sophisticated apparatus. With the additional finding of a raised intraocular pressure, glaucoma must be considered even if the optic disc appears relatively normal, as in this case. Where the colour is good, there is a healthy neuroretinal rim and only a slight nasal shift of the vessels. The degree of cupping might be normal. The early detection of glaucoma is very important, if further visual loss is to be avoided.

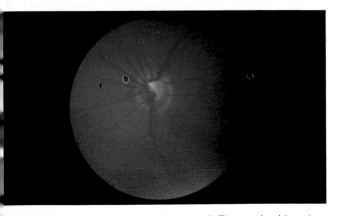

Fig.154 Glaucomatous cupping (advanced). The cup is widened and deepened; the disc is pale with a greenish hue. The blood vessels are shifted nasally and neural tissue at the rim of the cup is lost. Note how the temporal vessels disappear from view behind the overhanging edge. This is an advanced case and all visual field has been lost.

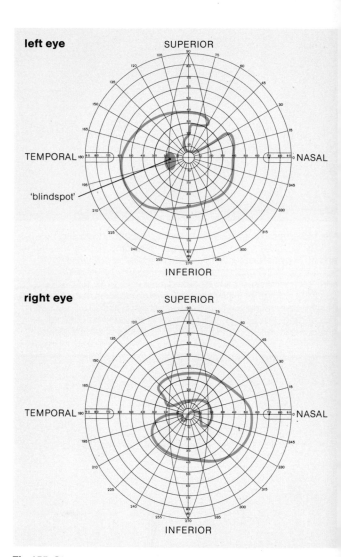

Fig.155 Glaucoma: field test. The fields shown here are from a patient with moderately advanced glaucoma. There is a scotoma ('arcuate') affecting the visual field in the left eye. This defect is more pronounced in the right eye and has advanced to meet the blind spot. Such asymmetry is usual. Failure to treat will lead to extinction of the field of vision. Treatment is aimed at reducing the intraocular pressure to a level where further deterioration of the fields is halted.

Index

All entries refer to Fig.
numbers